INFERTILITY AND ASSISTED CONCEPTION

WHAT YOU SHOULD KNOW

ANSWERS TO QUESTIONS ABOUT MEDICAL TECHNIQUES OF ASSISTED CONCEPTION

AGNETA SUTTON

THE CATHOLIC BISHOPS' JOINT COMMITTEE
ON BIO-ETHICAL ISSUES
London 1993

Published by
The Catholic Bishops' Joint Committee
on Bio-Ethical Issues

Distributed by
The Linacre Centre
60 Grove End Road
London NW8 9NH

British Library Cataloguing in Publication Data

Sutton, Agneta
 Infertility and Assisted Conception:
 What You Should Know
 I. Title
 176
 ISBN 0–9520923–0–1

Photoset & printed by
Redwood Press Ltd, Melksham, Wiltshire

Contents

		page
	Acknowledgements	iv
	Preface	v
	Introduction	1
Chapter 1:	Infertility and its treatment	3
Chapter 2:	When does an individual human life begin?	21
Chapter 3:	The moral issues	24
Chapter 4:	Prevention, cures and permissible forms of assisted conception	41
	Glossary	49
	Notes	55

Acknowledgements

I am grateful to all the members of the Catholic Bishops' Joint Committee on Bio-ethical Issues for their helpful comments on earlier drafts of this document. I am especially grateful to the Director of the Linacre Centre, Mr Luke Gormally, for his detailed comments on the final draft and to Bishop Christopher Budd, Dr John McLean, Bishop Donal Murray and the late Dr John Verzin for their critical reading of the first draft. Mgr Michael Connelly, Fr George Donaldson, Professor Peter Millard and Bishop Owen Swindlehurst very kindly provided helpful comments on the penultimate draft.

Finally, I wish to thank Dr Peter Doherty and Professor John Finnis – neither of whom are members of the Catholic Bishops' Joint Committee on Bio-ethical issues – for helpful comments relating to particular issues in the document.

Agneta Sutton

Preface

On the face of it developments in medicine designed to help people overcome distressing problems of infertility look as if they are entirely well-intentioned. But good ends need to be secured by good means – by means which respect human dignity and are themselves consistent with human well-being.

In this short book Agneta Sutton offers help to all those, and especially Catholics, who confront problems of infertility and who are anxious to find forms of medical assistance which both respect their dignity as potential parents and respect the dignity of the child they hope for.

The book provides a clear picture of the kinds of technical assistance in achieving conception which are on offer nowadays and the recognised medical risks of those techniques. But more importantly the book provides the guidance people need to determine which techniques are morally acceptable and which techniques are not.

In composing this book at the request of the Catholic Bishops' Joint Committee on Bioethical Issues, Agneta Sutton has worked collaboratively with it. The Committee which, apart from its episcopal members, contains experts from the fields of clinical medicine, nursing, biomedical research, the law, philosophy and theology, has had the opportunity of discussing various drafts of the book. We are extremely grateful for Agneta Sutton's collaboration in this enterprise and for the generous spirit in which she undertook the task of writing alongside her other commitments as Deputy Director of The Linacre Centre. Her contribution to the work of the Committee is one further example of the debt we owe to the staff of The Linacre Centre who have provided extensive help for the work of the Committee over the past decade.

Our essential task as a Committee, in face of the challenges posed by developments in modern medicine, has been that of discerning which practices are consistent with respect for human dignity and well-being and which practices (however well-intentioned) subvert human dignity and well-being. Agneta Sutton's book is a valuable contribution to that task in relation to medical developments designed to alleviate those problems of infertility which have come to afflict a significant percentage of people in our society.

Thomas J Winning
Archbishop of Glasgow
Chairman of The Catholic Bishops' Joint Committee
on Bioethical Issues.

Introduction

The Bible tells the story of Sarah and Abraham and their joy when, after many years of childlessness and despite Sarah's great age, she gave birth to a son, Isaac. 'God has given me cause to laugh', she said, and 'all who hear about this will laugh with me' (Gen. 21:6). St Luke's Gospel tells of another mother, Elizabeth, who was overjoyed to find herself pregnant after many years of longing for a child.

Today too there are many people who suffer because they cannot have children and who would be immensely grateful for a remedy. Modern medicine is able to treat many types of infertility which could not have been treated in the past. Such progress in medicine is welcome, but only provided the techniques employed respect human rights and do not infringe human dignity.

There are several techniques of medically assisted conception available today. Most of these techniques raise important moral questions. In some cases babies are being conceived outside marriage, because couples are offered sperm or ova which have been donated by a third party. Often, the procedures involved mean that babies are conceived not through sexual intercourse but as the result of purely technical procedures. Lastly, a number of the techniques involve, directly or indirectly, the destruction of unborn human life. In short, techniques of medically assisted conception raise a number of fundamental moral issues; these concern, on the one hand, the nature and dignity of the union of man and woman in marriage and in one flesh, and, on the other, the status and rights of the born and unborn child. Furthermore, because of their far-reaching implications, these issues are of the utmost importance not only for the couples seeking fertility treatment and for any new life they may engender, but also for society at large, both present and future, and for each one of us individually.

The first chapter of this document provides factual information about the medical procedures involved in various forms of treatment currently available. There is then a chapter concerning the question of when an individual human life begins. The third chapter deals with the moral issues raised by the different treatments. Finally, the fourth chapter is about morally acceptable remedies. The arguments are based on beliefs fundamental to Catholic morality: life is a gift from God; each person is created in the image of God; each person, therefore, by virtue of the human nature derived from the creative act from which he took his origin, possesses the same fundamental rights. The fundamental rights relevant to our enquiry are: the right to life and physical integrity from the moment of conception; the right to be conceived and reared by parents who have entered a marital commitment.[1]

1

Infertility and its treatment

What are the main causes of infertility?

The reproductive life of a woman begins with puberty and ends at the menopause. Throughout these reproductive years a mature ovum (egg) is released each month from the ovaries at the time of ovulation. This occurs approximately mid-way between one menstrual period and the next or, more precisely, some 14 days before the next expected period. At ovulation the ovum is picked up by the fallopian tube and it is in the fallopian tube that fertilisation normally takes place. If fertilisation does not occur within 12 hours of ovulation, the ovum will die and menstruation follows 12–14 days later. However, given the longer survival time of the sperm, intercourse four or five days before ovulation can result in fertilisation. This means that a woman is fertile for about five or six days each month: four or five days before ovulation plus one day after. But fertilisation is most likely if intercourse takes place around the time of ovulation. When fertilisation does take place, the embryo takes about 3–4 days to travel down the fallopian tube to the uterus and begin implanting there.

'Infertility' is a vague term. Most couples who want a child and who have regular intercourse achieve a pregnancy within a few months, i.e. within less than half a year. But few doctors would describe a couple as involuntarily infertile unless they had failed to achieve a pregnancy within two years of commencing regular intercourse. About 15 per cent of couples have fertility problems.[2]

A distinction is made between primary and secondary infertility.

Primary infertility refers to the condition of patients who have never conceived.

Secondary infertility refers to the condition of patients who have previously conceived but are finding difficulty in achieving a further conception.

Either type of infertility could be brought about by any of the following causes (the causes mentioned here are those most commonly found in industrialized countries)[3]:

1. Blocked or defective fallopian tubes, preventing the ovum from entering the tube or obstructing the passage of either ova or sperm through the tubes. This is one of the most common causes of infertility – especially, of secondary infertility (15–30 per cent of all cases). The problem can sometimes be corrected by tubal surgery.[4]

2. The inability to produce either ova or sperm (or sufficient sperm). This kind of problem is the most frequent cause of infertility (some 20–40 per cent of cases). It is more likely to be a cause of primary infertility than of secondary infertility. In women, the inability to produce ova can sometimes be overcome by hormone treatment. But there is as yet no treatment to induce sperm production in men.[5]

3. Abnormal structure of the woman's cervix (the neck of the womb), which completely or partially prevents the sperm from reaching the normal site of fertilisation (the fallopian tube). Surgical procedures can sometimes correct the defect.

4. Immunological factors in either the man or the woman, i.e. antisperm antibodies either in the man's semen or in the mucus of the woman's reproductive tract, which render the sperm inactive, and so prevent the sperm (completely or

partially) from reaching the normal site of fertilisation. Hormone treatment can help in some cases.[6]

5. Endometriosis is another common cause of infertility, especially primary infertility. It is a condition in which some of the lining of the uterus (called endometrial tissue) is misplaced in the woman's pelvis. This occurs in 10 per cent or more cases of infertility. The condition is sometimes successfully overcome by hormone treatment.[7]

What are the different methods of assisted conception available today?

The methods of assisted conception most commonly used at present are the following:

- Artificial insemination by husband – AIH
- Artificial insemination by donor – AID
- In vitro fertilisation – IVF
- Gamete intrafallopian transfer – GIFT
- 'IVF-related procedures', principally:
  i. Pronuclear stage tubal transfer – PROST
  ii. Tubal embryo transfer – TEST

Before discussing each of these methods, some consideration should be given to a procedure which is common to a number of them.

Superovulation

Women undergoing IVF treatment, GIFT treatment or other IVF-related procedures will be given hormone treatment to stimulate the ovaries in order to produce several ova in the same menstrual cycle, rather than the one ovum normally produced. This procedure – superovulation, as it is called – is thought to increase the chances of establishing a pregnancy. However, the treatment often involves a number of medical risks both for the mother and for any resulting child.

It is important to distinguish ovarian stimulation which is intended to produce several ova (perhaps half a dozen or so) from ovarian stimulation designed to overcome *failure to produce any ova at all* or other ovulation problems when this stimulation is carefully regulated in order to reduce the risk of producing several ova and several resulting conceptions – and so, quite possibly, a triplet or even quadruplet pregnancy.

What are the main risks of superovulation?

● *the risks for the woman*

A number of risks to a woman's health are associated with drug-induced superovulation. One dangerous – if rare – side-effect is ovarian hyperstimulation resulting in increased production of hormones, especially oestrogen. This can lead to excess fluid collection in the chest and abdomen which may be fatal. Other side-effects are the development of cysts, blood coagulation problems, stroke, cardiac arrest, molar pregnancy (abnormal, non-fetal cell-development) and ovarian cancer.[8]

Moreover, in the case of IVF and GIFT and other IVF-related procedures, there is the additional risk, when a number of ova or embryos are transferred to the womb, that the woman becomes pregnant with more than one child with all the attendant complications that may entail.[9]

To avoid the risks attached to the birth of several children at the same time, 'selective reduction', that is abortion of one or several fetuses, has been offered to mothers in cases of multiple pregnancy. Though the procedure requires the mother's informed consent, what she would consent to involves the destruction of some of her unborn children and may additionally affect her physical and psychological well-being.

- *the risks for the child*

Superovulation treatment can alter the hormone balance in the woman, and that may in turn affect the lining of the womb and render it inhospitable to the embryo, causing early embryo loss. If, on the other hand, a pregnancy is normally established, despite advice not to have sexual intercourse during the treatment, there is the risk of a multiple pregnancy. There is, likewise, a risk of a multiple pregnancy if, after superovulation treatment in connection with IVF, GIFT or other IVF related procedures, several ova or fertilized embryos are transferred to the mother at the same time. For the unborn children a multiple pregnancy is associated with the risk of premature birth and low birth weight (i.e. birth weight of less than 2,500g). Low birth weight, in its turn, is associated with an increased risk of death and illness in infancy.[10]

Artificial insemination by husband

For what forms of infertility is AIH recommended?

AIH may be offered to couples with the following types of problem[11]:

- *on the part of the man*

1. Insufficient sperm (in normal intercourse) – a condition called 'oligospermia'.
2. Paraplegia (paralysis of the lower part of the body and both legs).

- *on the part of the woman*

1. Absence of cervical mucus, preventing the passage of sperm through the cervix.
2. Cervical mucus containing antisperm antibodies, rendering the man's sperm inactive.

3. Abnormal cervical structure, preventing the passage of sperm through the cervix.

What does AIH involve?

AIH is usually a simple procedure whereby the husband's semen is deposited in the wife's uterus by means of a syringe. The husband's semen containing the sperm is usually obtained by masturbation.

Are there any risks?

AIH is less invasive and less complicated – and also less costly – than other procedures. And, for these reasons, it is often preferred as a first option.

What is the success rate?

The overall pregnancy rate is about 20 per cent.[12]

Artificial insemination by donor

Under what circumstances might a couple – or a single woman – be offered AID?

Donor insemination is used mainly in case of male infertility. It may be offered to a couple when the man suffers from one or other of the following conditions:
    1. a severe deficiency in the number of sperm produced at intercourse (severe oligospermia);
    2. impaired or inactive sperm (asthenospermia);
    3. total absence of sperm (azoospermia).[13]
    Recourse to AID may also be suggested if the husband

suffers from a grave hereditary disorder, which he would pass on to the next generation if he were to father any children. In the latter case AID is not a form of infertility treatment but a means of selective reproduction, a eugenic measure.

Finally, AID can be used by single women or, indeed, by lesbian couples, who seek to have a child without sexual contact with a man.

What does AID involve?

The insemination procedure is the same as in the case of AIH. The donor is screened specifically for transmissible diseases such as AIDS, syphilis and hepatitis B. The semen specimen is usually preserved for about six months so that the donor can be retested before it is used. Retesting is necessary for some conditions such as AIDS which may not be detected on the basis of a single test. In addition, the donor's blood group will be determined and his general health and medical history will be investigated.[14] Probably, a number of his physical characteristics will be recorded in order to ensure a fairly close match between his physical profile and that of the woman's husband. However, in the UK, as in most other countries, no identifying information is provided to the recipient(s).

A child born as the result of AID will have not one but two fathers: a genetic father (the donor) and a social or rearing father (normally, the mother's husband).

What are the risks?

In the past a few women have been infected with AIDS as a result of donor insemination. It is possible that the child too could contract the disease if the mother is infected from the donor. Conscientious screening of donors will minimize these risks but cannot rule them out altogether. Also, even if donors are carefully selected and screened, it is possible that a donor (whether he is aware of it or not) may pass on a grave hereditary disease to the children he fathers.

What is the success rate?

The pregnancy rate with AID is about 66 per cent when fresh semen is used and about 41 per cent with frozen semen.[15] This high success rate is to be explained by the fact that usually neither the donors nor the women involved are subfertile or infertile.

In vitro fertilisation

The term '*in vitro* fertilisation' – IVF for short – means fertilisation in a glass dish (hence *in vitro*, from the latin word *vitrum*, 'glass'). By contrast, normal fertilisation inside a woman is called fertilisation *in vivo* (a Latin phrase meaning 'in the living flesh').

Under what circumstances might a woman be offered IVF?

IVF is mainly a way of overcoming female infertility and may be offered under the following circumstances[16]:

1. Blockage or malfunction of the fallopian tubes. Often the women suffering from this condition have already undergone unsuccessful surgery with a view to correcting the tubal damage.

2. When for some reason both fallopian tubes have been removed.

3. In the case of defective entry of sperm into the uterus or the tubes, due either to:

(i) abnormal structure of the cervix (the neck of the womb) or the uterus, or to

(ii) the presence of antibodies in the cervical mucus.

4. Couples suffering from unexplained infertility may also be offered IVF. Interestingly enough, however, it has been observed that many such couples conceive while they are awaiting treatment.

In addition, in the future, single or lesbian women might seek IVF treatment with a view to achieving pregnancy without sexual contact with a man.

What are the procedures involved in IVF?

IVF usually involves the following procedures[17]:

- Superovulation to stimulate the woman's ovaries to produce several ova simultaneously, as opposed to the single one she would normally produce in one month.
- After superovulation, these ova are removed from the woman's ovaries.
- Semen is obtained from the woman's husband or partner – or from a donor.
- Each ovum is placed with sperm in a glass dish.
- If a number of ova are fertilised there will be several embryos.
- The embryos are examined under a microscope and 'healthy' ones are selected.
- The selected embryos, not more than three, are transferred to the uterus (usually the uterus of the woman providing the ova, but it could be the uterus of another woman) in the hope that at least one of them will implant in the lining of the uterus and develop successfully to be born nine months later.[18]
- 'Spare' embryos may be frozen and stored for later use by the couple (or woman). They may be donated to another couple or they may be used for research and then be destroyed. Other embryos not used for research may just be left to perish.

How are the ova 'harvested'?

In order to increase the chances of establishing a pregnancy it is common to place not one but two or three embryos into the uterus of the woman. This is why the first step in the IVF procedure is superovulation treatment to promote the ripening of several follicles in the ovaries so that up to half a dozen ova can be collected at the same time.

The most commonly used method of collecting the ova is by means of a needle which is passed, under the guidance of ultrasound scanning, into the ovary by way of the vagina. This technique has the advantage that it requires local anaesthesia only and not general anaesthesia.

Another method is the laparoscopic technique, which involves passing a thin tube through the wall of the abdomen and observing the ovaries while collecting the ova. Because this is a more invasive technique it requires general anaesthesia. This technique is now used less frequently than the ultrasound technique.

Is anything done to the sperm?

The semen has to be specially prepared in order to fertilise the ova. Certain proteins need to be washed from the surface of the sperm in order to enable the sperm to penetrate the wall of the ovum. Under normal circumstances when fertilisation takes place *in vivo*, the sperm are 'prepared' for fertilisation inside the female body.

What happens in the test-tube or petri-dish?

Each ovum is mixed separately with sperm in a test-tube or, more commonly, in a flat petri-dish. Fertilisation takes place and the embryos are closely observed to check that they are normal. Noticeably abnormal embryos will not be transferred to the uterus of the woman. The embryos are incubated in some cases for no more than four to sixteen hours but in other cases for up to two days or so before being transferred to the uterus.

How are the embryos transferred to the uterus of the woman?

The transfer procedure simply involves inserting the embryos (probably three) into the uterus by way of the vagina and through the cervix. This usually takes place on the second day (40–48 hours) after fertilisation.

What are the risks for the mother?

For the mother there are a number of risks attached to IVF.[19]

1. There are the risks attached to superovulation. Indeed, because of the serious risks attached to this procedure, some centres in the United States and France have now ceased to use it. It is noteworthy that several studies have reported success rates for IVF without superovulation which were no lower than for IVF in conjunction with superovulation.[20]

2. There is an increased risk of tubal pregnancy, which is dangerous.

3. There are also a certain number of risks attached to the surgical collection of ova.

4. In addition, any high-technology fertility treatment such as IVF, which is intrusive, painful and time consuming, may be accompanied by anxiety and other psychological side-effects. And, of course, IVF *does not cure* infertility but merely bypasses it. Moreover, if it is unsuccessful, as it is in some 90 per cent of cases, the patients are likely to experience a sense of failure, loss and grief as well as, quite possibly, anger and depression.[21] And if the woman undergoes 'selective reduction', her psychological well-being may be further affected by the knowledge of the killing that has taken place in her womb and her own involvement in it.

5. Finally, in those cases where IVF involves sperm donation, there are the risks of transmitting infectious disease to mother and child as well as of passing on an unsuspected hereditary condition to the child.

What are the risks for the embryo/child?

As a result of superovulation the woman usually produces six or more ova. But at most three embryos will be transferred to the womb. Thus since all the ova will probably be fertilised there will be surplus embryos. And this means that:

1. Many embryos are doomed to perish because they will never be transferred to the womb. They may be used for research (involving their destruction) or simply discarded. Advocates of IVF argue that further improvement of the technique requires various types of embryo research.

2. Other embryos will be frozen for future use. Unfortunately, however, many embryos are lost as a result of the practice of freezing surplus embryos for transfer to the woman at a later date in another treatment cycle.

3. In the future, embryo biopsy is likely to be a major cause of embryo wastage. At present many efforts are being made to develop techniques of embryo biopsy for diagnosis of hereditary illnesses prior to placing the embryo in the uterus. This is in order to 'weed out' embryos affected by hereditary – and other – disorders. In addition, employment of the technique will involve the loss of a number of healthy embryos as the procedure will not be risk-free. Yet there are many who hope that one day this technique will serve to replace much prenatal diagnosis and abortion on grounds of fetal abnormality carried out subsequent to implantation.[22]

Successfully transferred IVF embryos face other dangers.

4. Though normally conceived embryos may fail to implant, the failure rate of IVF embryos to implant is in excess of normal rates of failure. In many cases this is due to the

hormone treatment the woman received in order to stimulate superovulation.[23]

5. IVF is also associated with an increased risk of miscarriage later on in pregnancy.[24]

6. Tubal pregnancy is another danger.

7. When several embryos are transferred simultaneously, there is an increased risk of multiple pregnancy and low birth weight. Indeed, even when a woman is pregnant with only one child as a result of IVF, there is an increased risk of low birth weight and, as a consequence, the mortality rate among newly-born IVF babies is about four times as great as that among babies conceived normally.[25]

8. It has also been observed that the incidence of spina bifida among IVF babies may be as much as five times as great as the average. And the incidence of a certain type of congenital malformation of the heart may be as much as six times as great among IVF babies as among the general population of babies.[26]

What is the success rate?

The overall success rate of IVF is low. The method overcomes childlessness in about 10 per cent of patients undergoing the treatment.[27]

How many parents might the IVF baby have?

In most cases of IVF the man and the woman who provide the gametes (sperm and ova) are a married couple and the embryos are transferred to the uterus of the woman. The child, if there is one, is born to them and is genetically theirs. It has two parents: a mother and a father.

However, if for some reason the man is incapable of providing the sperm, the couple might be offered donated sperm for the treatment. Couples may also be offered donated sperm for eugenic reasons if the man suffers from a grave hereditary illness. When the sperm have been provided by a donor, the child will have not one but two fathers. It will have a genetic father, whose identity it will probably never know, since the law in this country (as in most others) protects the anonymity of the donor. Secondly, it will have a social or rearing father.

Another situation involving a male donor may arise if the woman is single and wishes to bear a child without sexual contact with a man. As the law stands at present, this situation is quite licit.[28] The child born through such an arrangement would have a mother, of course, and an unknown father, the donor.

There is also the possibility that a couple seeking IVF treatment may wish to have recourse to a female donor. The woman might be incapable of supplying the ova, although she is capable of carrying a child and of giving birth. Alternatively, the couple may be fertile, but the woman may be suffering from a genetic illness, which she and her partner do not wish to pass on to a child. A child born with the help of a female donor would have one father and two mothers. The donor mother, whom the child would not know, would be the genetic mother, while the gestational mother who would give birth would be the social and rearing mother.

IVF could also be used in connection with surrogacy arrangements. For medical or even social reasons, a man and a woman who want a child that is genetically theirs may hire the womb of another woman for gestation. A child born as the result of such an arrangement would have three parents: one father and two mothers. Besides its genetic mother (who intends to be its social mother) it would have a gestational mother (the mother who had been pregnant and bore the child), whom it might never get a chance to know. This differs from the more common type of surrogacy arrangement in which the surrogate mother is inseminated with sperm provided by the male party of the commissioning couple. In this case the genetic mother is also the gestational mother but will not be the social mother.

Other more complicated situations may arise using IVF. At the limit, the child could have five parents. There could be three different mothers: a genetic mother, a gestational mother and a social mother; and two fathers: a genetic father and a social father.

Gamete intrafallopian transfer (GIFT)

Under what circumstances might a couple – or a single woman – be offered GIFT?

Gift is a new technique which may be used provided the woman has at least one functioning fallopian tube. It may be offered in the following kinds of circumstance[29]:
1. the woman has endometriosis.
2. the woman's cervical mucus contains antisperm antibodies.
3. the cause of infertility is unknown.
4. donor insemination has failed.

What does GIFT involve?

Unlike IVF, GIFT does not involve embryo transfer, but the transfer of gametes (ova and sperm) to the woman. And these are transferred to the fallopian tube, not to the uterus. However, as in the case of IVF, GIFT usually involves super-ovulation. Usually two or three ova are transferred to the fallopian tube at the same time.

In GIFT the retrieval of ova and the transfer of ova and sperm to the fallopian tube are performed during the same operation by means of the laparoscopic technique, a procedure involving general anaesthesia. Occasionally, the ova may be retrieved either by a combination of laparoscopy and the ultrasound needling technique. The two (sometimes three) ova, separated by a small air bubble from sperm (obtained some two hours earlier), are then transferred to the tube.

What happens to spare ova?

Due to super-ovulation, more ova may be retrieved than can be used on one occasion for the purpose of establishing a pregnancy. These ova could be donated to another couple. Alternatively, they could be fertilised and frozen in order to be used for IVF, should the GIFT procedure prove unsuccessful. Other embryos might be used for research.

What are the risks for mother and child(ren)?

The risks for the women are much the same as in the case of IVF. In other words, there are the risks attached to the super-ovulation regime as well as those attached to the surgical procedures. The risks to the child are also much the same as in IVF.

What is the success rate?

The success rate of GIFT is of the same order as that of IVF.[30]

How many parents may be involved?

GIFT may involve donated sperm, but not usually donated ova. This is because with GIFT it is difficult to guarantee anonymity between donor and recipient, as both women have to be in hospital at the same time. Hence, the child would not normally have more than one mother but could well have two fathers: a genetic father (the donor) and a rearing or social father (the husband of the mother).

Pronuclear tubal transfer (PROST) and tubal embryo transfer (TEST)

What is the difference between PROST and TEST?

Both procedures involve embryo transfer to the fallopian tubes. They developed as modifications of GIFT in order to establish whether fertilisation has actually occurred.[31] In PROST the transfer of embryos to the fallopian tube takes place soon after fertilisation, before the first cell-division. (By 'fertilisation' is here meant penetration of the ovum by a sperm.) The retrieval of ova and the transfer of embryos are coordinated to take place one day after the other.

In TEST the embryos are transferred at a later stage when they consist of a few cells, and so the transfer takes place some time after the retrieval of ova. The embryos may even be frozen, allowing a further lapse of time between the retrieval of ova and the transfer of the embryo. Because there is no need to coordinate retrieval of ova and embryo transfer, TEST is more suitable than PROST in situations of ovum donation.

Under what circumstances might a couple be offered PROST or TEST?

PROST or TEST might be offered, for example, in case of male infertility when the woman's fallopian tubes are functional.

What do PROST and TEST involve?

Like all IVF-related procedures, PROST and TEST normally involve superovulation. Ova may be retrieved by means of the ultrasound technique by way of the vagina, in which case the procedure does not require general anaesthesia (*see* section on retrieval of ova in IVF, entitled *How are the ova 'harvested'?*). The transfer of embryos to the fallopian tube is performed, as in GIFT, by the laparoscopic technique and involves general anaesthesia. Spare ova may be donated or used for research or fertilized for future use involving IVF should the procedure fail.

Since both PROST and TEST might involve donation of both sperm and ova, a resulting child could, at the limit (as in the case of IVF), have five parents.

What are the risks and success rates?

The risks are obviously much the same as in IVF and GIFT. And the success rates too appear to be comparable.[32]

2

When does an individual human life begin?

When does an individual human life begin? There is only one reasonable answer to this question, namely: at fertilisation.

What, then, is accomplished at fertilisation?

With the exception of red blood cells, every cell in the human body has a nucleus – a centre – in which there are 46 chromosomes arranged in 23 pairs. These chromosomes carry the genes which are the biological basis of heredity. When the gametes (sperm and ovum) are formed, the chromosomal content of both sperm and ovum is reduced to 23 single chromosomes. Therefore, when the sperm penetrates the ovum at fertilisation, the embryo then formed has 46 chromosomes. And as the embryo develops and cell-division occurs, each new cell produced also has 46 chromosomes.

Once a sperm has penetrated an ovum at fertilisation, a new being has come into existence with intrinsic powers and potentialities different in kind from those of the two gametes taken separately. It is only because it has these special powers and potentialities that it can grow into a mature member of the species *homo sapiens*. Provided its development is not hampered by illness, accident or intentional destruction, it will achieve maturity and develop those abilities which are characteristic of mature human beings. From the very beginning the embryo has within itself the power to do so.

When does the life of the human individual begin?

Individual human life begins at fertilisation. This is because the difference between the day-old or hour-old embryo and the human adult is one of degree of maturity only, not of essential nature; the adult is a mature member of the species, whereas the embryo is a human person whose characteristic human powers and potentialities have only just begun to be developed and actualized. From the time of conception onwards the development of the human being is gradual and continuous. Thus, although the embryo does not yet look like a child and possesses none of the special abilities typical of mature human beings, it is already an actual human being, not a potential one.

This may seem a statement of the obvious. For, surely, every adult knows that he or she was once a child and takes it for granted that he or she was once a fetus and a newly-formed embryo. And, surely, every person also takes it for granted that at each stage of growth and development he or she was the same being as he or she is today.

Yet there are those who say that this cannot be true. They argue, for instance, that sometimes the embryo 'twins' and becomes, not one, but two individual human beings. This shows (they go on to argue) that individual human life cannot begin until the embryo has reached the stage at which it is no longer possible for it to twin. And this stage is reached, they conclude, only at about fourteen days after fertilisation.

What is disputable is the assumption that, because *some* embryos twin, *all* embryos have an active tendency to twin. The evidence we have about twinning does not support this assumption. There is a fairly standard incidence of monozygotic twinning across all human populations (about 0.03 per cent of live births[33]). This is one fact which suggests that the active tendency to twin is genetically determined and is peculiar to a very small percentage of embryos.

If the active tendency to twin is peculiar to a very small percentage of embryos, then the first thing we can say is that twinning provides no clear objection to regarding the vast majority of embryos as individual human beings from fertilisation. Secondly, we can say about an embryo which does twin that if it is programmed from the start to become two individual beings, then two lives are, in a sense, already present in it.

Another reason why some people hold that the early embryo is not an individual being – and, therefore, that it cannot be identified with the later fetus, the child and the adult – is that only some of the cells of the early embryo will develop into the fetus, while others will come to form the placenta and other extra-embryonic tissue such as the umbilical cord and the amniotic sac, i.e. the bag of waters. However, the fact that some of the early embryonic cells are precursors of the placenta does not disprove but rather testifies to the embryo's organic unity from the start. That the placenta is developed precisely as an organ which is, for a time, necessary for the support of early human life shows the single goal-directedness which underlies the differentiation and development of early embryonic life. It is a manifestation of the functional unity of the organism right from the start. And the fact that the placenta is lost at the birth of the child has no more bearing on its individuality than does the loss of the child's milk-teeth at a later stage in its life. In other words, the fact that only some of the cells forming part of the early embryo will develop into fetal tissue does not prove that the early embryo is not an individual being.

Everything we know about the development of the embryo testifies to the fact that at fertilisation there comes into being a new human individual, that is, a person.

3

The moral issues

If, as has been shown, individual human life or the life of a person begins at the time of conception (fertilisation), then from that time onwards what has been conceived deserves our respect and possesses human rights as do other members of the human family. Above all the conceptus possesses the same right to life as any one of us. Some people find it hard to see that individual human life, personal life, begins at conception; they cannot bring themselves to believe that the conceptus, given its appearance, is really a human being. But although the characteristic powers and potentialities of the human embryo have only just begun to develop and actualise, it is precisely that process of development which leads, without discontinuity, to human maturity. And because human life is continuous from the time of fertilisation it should be understood and treated as a totality at all stages from that time onwards. Thus to cut short a human life in the bud is to shorten the totality of the life of a man-to-be or of a woman-to-be. It is to cut short the life of a person.

Because of this, assisted conception raises three morally important questions:

1. Are the methods of assisted conception described above compatible with the right to life of human embryos and

fetuses and with their right not to be exposed intentionally to the risk of severe harm?

2. Do those who take part in those methods of assisted conception offend against the human dignity of the young person, the child born as a result of these techniques?

3. Are those methods of assisted conception in keeping with the dignity of the parents and the institution of marriage?

The arguments below are based on beliefs and reasoning fundamental to Catholic morality. The most recent pronouncement by the Catholic Church on these issues is *Donum Vitae* or, as it is called in English, *Instruction on Respect for Human life in Its Origin and on the Dignity of Procreation: Replies to Certain Questions of the Day*, issued by The Congregation for the Doctrine of the Faith in 1987. And the conclusions reached here are in accord with those to be found in that document.

Assisted conception and the risks to the mother and the unborn child

Is superovulation morally acceptable?

Hormone stimulation to induce ovulation or to overcome ovulation problems is morally acceptable if the intention is to help the woman's body to function normally and if the procedure is carefully regulated so as to avoid overstimulation or the production of several ova in the same menstrual cycle. In this case the treatment is a cure restoring the woman to bodily health, and so giving her a chance to reproduce through ordinary sexual intercourse within marriage.

But superovulation in connection with IVF and GIFT and other IVF related procedures, in which the intention is to produce several ova (up to half a dozen) at the same time, is unethical. It exposes the mother to serious risks (*see* Chapter 1, section on superovulation, subsection entitled *The risks for the woman*). And if the woman becomes pregnant while undergoing this treatment, there is the risk of a multiple pregnancy.

This is also the case if, after superovulation in connection with IVF or GIFT or other related procedures, several ova or embryos are transferred to the mother at the same time. For the unborn children a multiple pregnancy is associated with the risks of miscarriage or premature birth. And premature birth, in its turn, is associated with an increased risk of death or illness in infancy.

Respect for the life of the unborn would be further undermined if the medical team with the consent of the couple were to carry out 'selective reduction' of a multiple pregnancy, that is the abortion of one or more of the fetuses with a view to reducing their number.

In what other ways do IVF, GIFT, PROST and TEST violate the embryo's right to life?

As we have seen, IVF and related procedures normally involve the production of many more embryos than can be transferred to a woman on one occasion. Some of the surplus or 'spare' embryos may be frozen and transferred to the womb on a later occasion. Many will be used for research purposes, while others will be left to perish. The situation is similar in the case of GIFT. For here too usually more ova are produced than can be used on one occasion and these surplus ova may be fertilised and treated as other 'spare' embryos.

As for the selection procedure in connection with embryo transfer (in IVF, PROST and TEST), the healthiest looking ones will, of course, be picked out and given a chance to develop into mature human beings. At present the procedure is a rather crude one based on observation of the embryos under the microscope. But with the development of embryo biopsy it will become possible to find out whether a particular embryo suffers from a genetic (hereditary) disease, or some other condition or characteristic which is considered undesirable. Despite the risk that the procedure itself might destroy the embryo, pre-implantation diagnosis and eugenic embryo selection are set to become part and parcel of IVF and related techniques in the future. Moreover, such techniques will not be confined to patients who have sought fertility treatment. Parents-to-be naturally want healthy children. With the availability today of prenatal diagnosis and selective abortion (of defective fetuses), many parents who would not otherwise have attempted pregnancy now do so in the knowledge that the pregnancy can be terminated if the child is found to be affected by an abnormality. The day that pre-implantation diagnosis by means of embryo biopsy becomes widely available, many people will undoubtedly consider this a more humane way of assisting couples than the present practice of offering prenatal diagnosis with termination in case of fetal abnormality.

But if human embryos and fetuses already are human beings, neither abortion nor pre-implantation selection can be justified. Killing by pre-implantation selection of embryos and killing by selective abortion are both equally unacceptable. Both are ways of weeding out certain human beings.

Furthermore, both prenatal diagnosis and pre-implantation diagnosis expose those who are tested to serious risks of harm. But embryos and fetuses, since they are human beings, have the same basic rights as the rest of us; which means that it is wrong not only to kill them outright, but even to expose them to serious risk of death or grave injury.

For this very reason the practice of freezing embryos must also be rejected as wrong, since many embryos perish as a result of this procedure.

The most abhorrent practice of all in connection with IVF and similar procedures is the use of human embryos in research involving their destruction. To undertake such research is to treat members of our own species as mere disposable material or tissue. The embryos subjected to experimentation are, as we have seen, either 'spare embryos' left over after IVF and other related treatments or embryos specifically produced for research purposes from spare ova. These ova, in turn, may have been left over from such treatments or they may have been obtained from those hysterectomies which involve the removal of one or both ovaries.

In conjunction with IVF and related techniques, then, human embryos are being deliberately created in order to be subjected to experiments which can only harm and kill them. This is said to be justified because such experiments may be to the advantage of other human beings. It is argued that such experiments will lead to new and better ways of treating infertility and, through the development of pre-implantation diagnosis, to healthier babies. It is also said that such experiments will produce new means of contraception. The answer to this is that we are all created in the image of God and so have an equal right to life and protection. Hence, it is never justified to treat a human being as a mere means and to sacrifice him or her for the good of others.

Because all human beings have an equal right to life, all human embryos – since they are human beings – have an equal right to life irrespective of the circumstances of their conception. It makes no difference whether they have been conceived for a purpose which in itself is good or whether conception has taken place inside or outside the body of a woman, or whether the embryos have been conceived with or without medical assistance. To quote from *Donum Vitae*:

> Human embryos obtained *in vitro* are human beings and subjects with rights: their dignity and right to life must be respected from the first moment of their existence. *It is immoral to produce human embryos destined to be exploited as disposable 'biological material'.* (*Donum Vitae*, Part I, para. 5).

In short, inasmuch as the IVF, PROST, TEST and GIFT techniques involve the risk of causing grievous harm to embryonic human life, and insofar as the development of the techniques depend on the intentional destruction of embryos in research, these techniques constitute a grave injustice towards the very youngest and smallest members of our species.

Assisted conception and the dignity of the child

Can one say that people have a right to have a child?

Husband and wife, having committed themselves to a shared life, have a right to enjoy the marital act and to care for the fruit of that act. That is to say, a man and a woman who have entered a marital commitment have a right to *seek* to have a child, provided they do so in a way consistent with that commitment and consistent with the dignity of the child. But no one has the right to *obtain* a child because no one can have a duty to provide them with a child. Nor could any doctor ever promise them a child even if he wanted to help them. No matter what a couple is prepared to pay to have a child and no matter what trouble their doctor is willing to go to, not even the best doctor in the best clinic in the world could promise them a child at the end of the day. In skilled hands, they may have one if God permits. That is all!

The marital vow is a vow to be faithful; to have children within marriage only and to bring them up within marriage. When this is the case the child is conceived through the sexual act in the context of a stable relationship based on a firm commitment.

The father and the mother of the child do not make it. But they receive it in giving themselves to each other in their sexual embrace. The child is a gift – a very special gift. Because it is begotten, not made, of one being with its parents, it is flesh of the parents' flesh and, therefore, their equal as a human being. Like its parents, the child is a person created in the image of God. It possesses the same human dignity as its parents and must be treated with the respect due to every human being.

Today, however, many people see a child as something which one decides to have or not to have, in the way that one decides to buy or not to buy a car. They think they have a right to a child because they are inclined to view the child as a chattel rather than as a person. They fail to recognise its human dignity and its human rights. But, human beings simply are equals, created in the image of God, begotten not made. They cannot own one another. Children are not possessions.

Why is the child wronged if it is brought into the world by means of assisted conception which bypasses normal intercourse?

Infertility is a misfortune. But a couple's very understandable desire for a child does not justify their seeking to have a child at all costs. It is perhaps not surprising that many who think they have a right to a child also think that any medical intervention which may make that possible is justified. But certain methods of assisted conception offend against the dignity of the child by treating it as if it were a mere product and property. This, in fact, is true of all forms of assisted conception, except those which facilitate the natural process of generation within marriage (*see* Chapter 4 on morally permissible forms of assisted conception).

What distinguishes morally justifiable methods from AIH, AID, GIFT, IVF and related procedures that do not involve the normal sexual act is that the former do not interfere with the natural process of generation in which conception takes place in the female body as the result of a man and a woman having sexual intercourse. That is to say, what makes most techniques now used unacceptable is that they do not facilitate the natural process but bypass it altogether. Procreation is separated from intercourse. Hence, the child is not begotten by a couple in or through their bodily union but is a product of the actions of third parties.

In the case of methods of assisted conception where the child's generation has nothing to do with the conjugal or sexual act the generation of the child is similar to the production of an artefact. This is especially true when the child is produced by means of highly technical procedures such as GIFT, IVF and related techniques. Here the child is the end-product of a great number of complicated procedures involving, amongst other things, the handling of gametes in laboratories by doctors, nurses and laboratory staff. Apart from the maternal gestation – no minor part, of course – the role of the parents is subordinated to that of the medical team. The medical team is in charge. Indeed, the child is theirs to the extent that it is the result of their achievements. But it is theirs not in virtue of an act expressive of love but rather in virtue of a technical mastery over biological 'materials'.

In short, methods of assisted conception which bypass the sexual act encourage the view that the child is a man-made product, an artefact. They dehumanise and so have a built-in tendency to degrade the child, however much people may strive to resist that tendency.

Why does a child have a right to be born within marriage?

Children need security. They need a stable home. Marriage is the institution most likely to provide that stability. The couple who take their marital commitment seriously see each other as non-substitutable partners for life. Couples who live together without a formal commitment to stay together cannot offer their children the same stability. They may intend to stay together but without a formal promise to do so it is easier for them to break up, should they be tempted to do so. And there is no doubt that lack of security in homes, marital break-ups and temporary unions have repercussions for the young and, indeed, for society at large. These things affect the lives of all the individuals concerned, the adults and the children. They affect their relationship to other people and the way they act at work or at school. Most important, they may affect the children's ability to form lasting and trusting relationships later on in life.

Only a promise of total commitment can prepare the couple for the responsibilities of parenthood which entail many years of caring for another human being and provision of a proper preparation for adulthood.

Why does the child have a right to be born as the true genetic child of its parents?

The implications of the marital vow in regard to the relationship between man and woman in their role as parents are discussed at greater length in the final section of the present chapter about the dignity of parenthood. Suffice it to say in this context that, because the marital vow implies faithfulness until death, it encourages a relationship of mutual trust, acceptance and oneness.

It is precisely this relationship of mutual trust, acceptance and oneness that is threatened by gametal donation. Married couples seeking fertility treatment find that assisted procreation involving gametal donation turns out to be a strain on their relationship rather than a unifying experience. Of course there is no question here of infidelity in the sense of one of the parties having engaged in extramarital sexual relations. But the acceptance of gametal donation amounts to a denial of the exclusiveness of the spousal relationship. And insofar as gametal donation separates rather than unifies the family, it clearly threatens not only the relationship between the parents but also their relationship with the child.

Besides the effects on the couple's marriage and the consequences of these for the child, the child born as a result of gametal donation risks suffering from identity problems. A child born as the result of sperm donation (which could be part of any of the procedures dealt with above except, of course, AIH) may well, if it knew the truth, ask itself questions about its genetic father. Similarly, in the case of ovum donation (which could accompany either IVF, PROST or TEST), the child may well wonder who its genetic mother was and what she was like. Indeed, this situation might be even more difficult to cope with than sperm donation. The child might feel emotionally split between, on the one hand, its gestational mother who gave it life by nourishing it within her own body for nine months and, on the other, the genetic mother who provided fifty percent of its hereditary make-up. Such situations are of their nature apt to cause both social and psychological problems for the child.

Many people argue, however, that if adopted children can cope with their situation, then so too can children born as the result of gametal donation. But adoption may cause identity problems, especially if the child never finds out who its genetic parents are. Moreover, there are several important differences between the two situations. Insofar as public records are available, the adopted child has a right to learn who its genetic parents are when it reaches the age of majority. This is not the case when the child has been generated by means of donation. The law protects the donor's right to anonymity, and so the child is legally prevented from gaining access to records that would shed light on that part of its parentage. All it will ever learn is a basic description of the main observable traits and characteristics of the donor such as his or her ethnic origin, the colour of his or her skin, hair and eyes, his or her blood group and the like. Moreover, it is one thing to adopt a child who is already there. This is to welcome an orphan into one's home. It is quite another matter to go out of one's way to bring a child into this world in such a way that it will be placed in a parentally ambiguous situation.

Another important consideration is the risk of incest. That is to say, there is the risk that children related by a common donor may later in adult life unwittingly marry or enter into a sexual relationship with each other.

In addition, gametal donation fosters procreational or parental irresponsibility on the part of donors. This consideration perhaps applies especially in the case of sperm donation since this can be so easily done. The proponents of gametal donation may picture it as a kind of generosity. But in regard to the child who is conceived it entails serious deprivation resulting precisely from dereliction of responsibility on the part of donors. Children have a special right not to be abandoned by their parents. The parental obligation to care for one's children is one of the most fundamental obligations of all. To join in begetting a child should be seen for the choice it properly is: a special commitment to meeting the developmental needs of that child in ways conducive to the child's eventual maturity. If human beings do not hold on to *this* understanding of what is involved in begetting a child then the consequences for children will be disastrous.

Donation could also have far-reaching effects on social attitudes towards the disabled and ill. This is because it could encourage selective reproduction favouring certain types of donor and offspring. In this case it could result in an increased intolerance and even rejection of children who do not live up to parental or social expectations.

Finally, even if many parents who have accepted gametal donation are very loving and excellent parents, by its nature gametal donation encourages a 'consumerist' attitude towards the child. For the couple who obtain or avail of gametes from a donor satisfy their desire for a child by a transaction which is – or resembles – a commercial transaction. Effectively, this reduces the child to an object that can be obtained in the market place. To treat a child thus, as a chattel, constitutes a grave failure to show it the proper respect it is owed as an equal member of the human family.

Why do certain 'quasi-family arrangements' (such as lesbian ones), rendered possible by gametal donation, violate the rights of the child?

Today there are single women who seek medical assistance not because they are infertile but in order to have a child without sexual contact with a man. The form of assisted reproduction they seek is usually artificial insemination by donor. But their wishes might also be fulfilled by means of IVF, GIFT or TEST.

Women may secure artificial insemination by donor by doing it themselves or with the help of their friends. The procedure is not complicated and semen could be obtained from male friends or indirectly, for the sake of anonymity, through third parties. It might even be obtained from sperm banks attached to fertility clinics; recourse to these centres would be advantageous because sperm would have been tested for AIDS and other transmissible diseases.

Deliberately to embark on the project of being a single mother is obviously wrong since this is aiming to deprive the child of a father. (Of course, most single mothers have become such without acting on the basis of any plan of that kind.)

Without both a father and a mother the child's future is less secure. In addition, the father and the mother complement one another. Human beings are created male and female. Together the two bring forth new life. Single women who have children through insemination deny this truth in practice by their way of life while admitting it in their act of accepting donation of male seed. This involves a suppression of truth and consequent self-deception. Moreover, the child growing up in an ordinary two-parent family learns something both from its father and its mother. It is being prepared for the normal commitments of family life and, quite generally, for an adult world containing both men and women. There can be no doubt that the social development of a child is furthered when the child is reared in a family where there is both a father and a mother.

Of course, it is not only female procreational irresponsibility that is at issue here. As pointed out above, donor insemination within marriage – as well as outside – encourages male procreational irresponsibility. It is an institutionally organised and sanctioned way of allowing a man to disown the child he fathers, the child whose genetic father he is and remains forever.

This does not mean that a single parent cannot do a very good job of bringing up a child alone if he or she has to because of bereavement, desertion or separation. However, single parents themselves are often keenly aware of the heroic efforts they may have to undertake and the enormous demands made on them in trying to bring up children on their own.

In short, for single women to resort to donor insemination or IVF-related techniques for the purpose of rearing a child is to do the child a triple injustice. It is to deny it a home based on marriage, to expose it to all the ills of gametal donation and to deprive it of a father.

As for lesbian couples who have children, they do them an even greater injustice. Not only do they deprive their children of a father and expose them to problems of gametal donation but, in addition, they place them in a situation which is a moral and social aberration. To help a lesbian couple to become 'parents' is to allow a child to become part of a set-up which cannot but fail to prepare it properly for adult life. The same applies, of course, to homosexual couples who adopt a child. Irrespective of how lavish the affection and care a single-sex couple give to a child, they place it in a situation where it will be morally, socially and psychologically deprived, if not disturbed, by the fact that both persons playing the role of 'parent' are of the same sex.

The dignity of parenthood

Why is the marital commitment of prime importance for a man and a woman in their vocation as parents?

As a social institution marriage entails a formal vow to be faithful and to share sorrows as well as pleasures. It is based on mutual trust, love, support and respect.

Furthermore, as a sacred institution, marriage is a non-dissolvable union because it makes husband and wife one before God. Marriage is a divine gift, both to man and woman as a couple and to human society. The sacrament of marriage entails exclusive and mutual self-giving until the end of life. It also entails openness to new life. That is to say, marriage is not only a relationship between a man and a woman but also between the couple and their Father in Heaven. The marriage celebrated in the Church is a promise to cooperate with God in the creation of new human life and in the loving care of the young. This means that human procreation is subject not only to human laws and mores but also to the divine law for our fulfilment.

By promising love and fidelity before God the couple prepare a haven for themselves and a home prepared to welcome children and bring them up in love and security. Moreover, by making each other non-substitutable, husband and wife undertake to become father and mother through each other only. And every child born to them becomes the incarnation of their exclusive and enduring love.

Without mutual support based on a sincere commitment men and women are ill-prepared for the responsibilities of parenthood. Not only does the child need a father and mother but, in addition, because the demands of parenthood are many and not always light, the father and the mother need each other. They need to share and they need to know that they can rely on each other. Perhaps the mother in particular needs to know that she can depend on her spouse. This is because she is the one who gives birth and cares for the very young. And so the man who loves and respects the mother of his children will want to give her his assurance of unfailing support. But fathers too need the love and security of a warm and caring home in order to face the demands of paternity. Just as every mother needs a caring and dependable husband, so too every father needs a caring and dependable wife.

Procreation outside marriage is not for the good either of the individual or society. Couples who live together outside marriage and who have children do themselves, their children and society at large an injustice by not sealing their relationship with the conjugal vow without which their relationship may be easy prey to human weaknesses. Similarly, women who decide to have children on their own without the complementarity and support of a husband fail to show true regard not only for their offspring but also for themselves. Marriage is the only true foundation of the family.

Why is gametal donation incompatible with the dignity of the spouses?

The marriage commitment of husband and wife to treat each other as irreplaceable is essential to the character of marriage. In so far as husband and wife treat each other as irreplaceable, their relationship is geared to secure oneness and trust – and so what is essential to the good of their children: the knowledge that they too are irreplaceable and are valued for precisely the persons they are.

The dignity of a spouse is respected only insofar as the spouse is treated as irreplaceable. But a husband whose wife has a child as a result of donor insemination is treated as someone who is replaceable, as is the wife whose husband produces a child with the help of a surrogate. This is partly true too of the wife who accepts ovum donation in order to bear a child for her husband and herself. It should come as no surprise to anybody if a spouse who has been replaced in the very act of procreation suffers diminished self-respect and in some way feels betrayed. Where is the unique intimacy and sharing normally accompanying the conception of a child?

This does not mean that people cannot adopt a child together because it is not theirs. And it does not mean that a widow with a child could not marry again because the new father would not be the genetic father of the child. There is an important difference between these situations and gametal donation. The couple who adopt a child take home a child who is already born. They truly share in their act of welcoming that child into the family. The arrival of this child is compatible with their conjugal vow of exclusive fidelity. And, since the conjugal vow is phrased 'until death do us part', the widow's second marriage is not a denial of her old vows; and the act of the man who opens his heart to her child is but an act of generosity.

Why do means of assisted conception which bypass the normal process of generation offend against the dignity of man and woman?

In IVF, GIFT, PROST and TEST, and in AID as well as AIH the sexual act is bypassed. But it is contrary to human dignity to separate procreation from the unitive aspect of physical love. People who resort to methods of assisted conception, which bypass the physical embrace and render it superfluous to the life-giving process of fertilisation, treat the child as an artefact and themselves as no more than providers of raw material from which it is manufactured. This is degrading for the child and it means a spiritual impoverishment for the man and the woman. The act of procreation is no longer the embodiment of their loving and spiritual union and their child is no longer received as a gift in the act of mutual self-giving but is a product of the manipulative industry of others.

Indeed, highly technical forms of fertility treatment such as IVF tend to make an object not only out of the child but also out of the couple, especially the woman. This is because others – doctors and nurses and laboratory technicians – take control over the most intimate aspects of the couple's life.

In short, methods of assisted conception which bypass the sexual embrace dehumanise man, woman and child. They constitute a denial of the fundamental meaning of that act, which through divine wisdom and by the laws of nature was ordained to constitute the sole means whereby new life should be given.

4

Prevention, cures and morally permissible forms of assisted conception

When God created human beings, so we read in the Bible, 'male and female He created them' and 'God blessed them saying to them, "Be fruitful, multiply, fill the earth and conquer it"' (Gen. 1. 27–28).

Sadly enough many people cannot live up to this injunction however dearly they may wish to do so. Infertility is a problem affecting a considerable proportion of people both in richer countries (about 14 per cent[34]) and in the poorer parts of the world (well over 20 per cent in some parts of Africa[35]).

The Church recognises the suffering caused by infertility and urges scientists and members of the medical profession to search for its causes and for ways of preventing and curing it. And, contrary to what many people seem to assume, the Church is not opposed to assisted conception, provided the means used respect the dignity of the human individual, that is, the human dignity of the child, the woman and the man. This view is clearly stated in *Donum Vitae*:

> Many researchers are engaged in the fight against sterility. While fully safeguarding the dignity of human procreation, some have achieved results which previously seemed unattainable. Scientists therefore are to be encouraged to continue their research with the aim of preventing the causes of sterility and of being able

to remedy them so that sterile couples will be able to procreate in full respect for their own personal dignity and that of the child to be born. (*Donum Vitae*, Part II, para. 8)

Can some forms of infertility be prevented?

In the poorer parts of the world infertility is often due to malnutrition and illness such as tuberculosis (which may cause blocked fallopian tubes).[36] In these parts, then, infertility could in many cases be avoided by better living conditions and, in particular, by better hygiene and an improved diet.

In many parts of the world, also, including both poorer and richer countries, a change in sexual mores would have a beneficial effect and prevent much infertility, notably infertility caused by venereal infection, especially in women. Blocked fallopian tubes, for instance, are commonly the result of infection caused by sexually transmitted diseases.[37]

Contraceptive measures may also cause infertility in women. Thus the IUD (intra-uterine device) which has been widely used both in the West and in developing countries such as India, is another leading cause of tubal infection and blocked tubes. But because of a number of undesirable side-effects, especially discomfort and excessively heavy menstrual periods, this device is now less popular in the United States and Europe than it was in the 1970s.

A third major cause of infertility is procured abortion.[38] Indeed, in the countries that used to make up the Soviet Union this could be the main cause of infertility.

The contraceptive pill, too, which has been most widely used in the West, may cause infertility for one or even two years after discontinuance. And this is in women who have previously been fertile, i.e., women who have had children.

Unfortunately, these matters are not widely discussed. And many people are ignorant of the possible side-effects of the drugs and devices they are being prescribed by doctors. Many people are even unaware of the main effects of these drugs and devices or of how they work. From the beginning the medical profession suspected that the IUD worked not solely as a contraceptive preventing fertilisation but as an abortifacient preventing implantation of newly-fertilised embryos. But the majority of patients who were fitted with the device were clearly not informed about this or about the distinction between, on the one hand, preventing fertilisation, and on the other, preventing implantation. And today it is known, at least among the members of the medical profession, that 'the pill' too, especially if it contains a lower hormone dosage (as these days the most widely prescribed varieties do) works partly as an abortifacient by preventing implantation.

Catholic doctors, nurses and midwives, as well as members of these professions who belong to other faiths and who respect unborn human life, have a special duty both to inform their individual patients about these facts and to speak up in public.

> It is only logical ... to address an urgent appeal to Catholic doctors and scientists that they bear exemplary witness to the respect due to the human embryo and to the dignity of procreation. The medical and nursing staff of Catholic hospitals and clinics are in a special way urged to do justice to the moral obligations which they have assumed ... (*Donum Vitae*, Part II, Para. 7)

It is as ironical as it is tragic that many young women in their twenties are being eagerly assisted by the medical profession in their efforts to avoid becoming pregnant, only to be obliged to seek further medical assistance in their thirties or forties in order to overcome infertility, when this problem has been caused precisely by the damage done to their reproductive system by their previous use of contraceptives, or by recourse to abortion.

In short, Catholic doctors and nurses have a special obligation to help their patients and the public to prevent certain kinds of infertility by providing information about preventable causes of this misfortune.

Are there morally acceptable cures for some kinds of infertility?

Unfortunately, not all infertility is preventable. Research into cures is, therefore, to be welcomed, provided it respects the dignity of the individuals involved and is not performed at the cost of sacrificing embryonic human life.

By 'cure' is here meant methods of overcoming infertility either surgically or with medical drugs in such a way that the individuals 'cured' thereafter can procreate unassisted through ordinary sexual intercourse. Cures, so understood, are morally acceptable. They make conception possible in a manner which respects the dignity both of the couple and of their prospective child.

There are a number of such possible cures, which can be considered in relation to different kinds of case.

The wife is incapable of producing ova

Hormone treatment may overcome infertility in women caused by failure to produce ova – thus allowing reproduction by ordinary sexual intercourse.

The couple are capable of producing gametes but are not achieving pregnancy.

Here several approaches are possible.

1. Surgery to correct tubal blockage and allow fertilisation to take place in the fallopian tube. The woman who has been successfully operated on can have babies without any further

medical assistance (*see* Chapter 1, section *What are the Main Causes of Infertility*).

2. Likewise, defective entry of sperm into the upper female reproductive tract caused by abnormal structure of the cervix or uterus can in some cases be corrected by surgical procedures.

3. Drug therapy (probably administration of hormones) can be employed to overcome impaired entry into the female upper reproductive tract caused by immunological factors, i.e., sperm anti-bodies (*see* Chapter 1, section *What are the Main Causes of Infertility*).

4. Endometriosis, or misplaced uterine lining, can often be successfully treated by drug therapy or surgery (*see* Chapter 1, section *What are the Main Causes of Infertility*).

Couples who have been cured by any of these procedures may not need further medical assistance in order for the woman to become pregnant. For them there is no question of separating procreation from sexual intercourse, since it is possible for them to conceive a child by ordinary intercourse.

Are there any morally acceptable forms of assisted conception?

Even if much research is undertaken into the causes of infertility with a view to prevention and cure, there are situations in which a real cure is not available and couples may need other forms of medical assistance in order to have children. The question arises, therefore, whether there are morally acceptable ways of helping such couples which respect their dignity by not separating procreation from the conjugal act. In other words, are there ways of assisting such couples which do not bypass the sexual act and render it superfluous? The answer is: Yes. For there are medical interventions which, as *Donum Vitae* puts it, simply 'assist the conjugal act either in order to facilitate its performance or to achieve its objective once it has been normally performed' (Para. II, 6) and thus allow the child to be 'the fruit of a specific act of conjugal union' (Para, II, 4).

Donum Vitae makes a distinction between, on the one hand, interventions which bypass sexual intercourse and amount to a substitute for it and, on the other, interventions which facilitate the performance of the sexual act, complete a process initiated by the sexual act or allow the sexual act to be causally effective in achieving conception.

Thus, if difficulties relating to the very performance of the sexual act were to be overcome by the help of medical assistance or technical means, this would be morally permissible inasmuch as it would assist the couple to perform the act in the natural manner and so conceive a child.

There are also ways of assisting couples, who would not otherwise conceive, to achieve fertilisation once the sexual act has been performed normally.

As AIH is commonly performed, it involves masturbation in order to obtain sperm. This means that the sexual act becomes superfluous. Fertilisation, if it is achieved, is achieved without coitus; the child is not begotten in or through the sexual embrace as befits the dignity of man, woman and child.

However, there is a procedure which in some respects resembles AIH but which is to be distinguished from it and which is performed in a manner that respects the dignity of the individual persons. Thus it is possible for a couple, after intercourse, to have recourse to medical assistance in order to transport sperm deposited in the vagina further up the female reproductive tract so that fertilisation can take place. This would be a morally acceptable way of helping a couple, if the wife's cervix did not allow the passage of sperm to the uterus.

This intervention does not constitute a substitute for the sexual act, as would be the case if the sperm were *removed* from the vagina and then, through a subsequent medical intervention reintroduced into the woman's body and deposited in her uterus or tubes for fertilisation. The sperm to be used in GIFT could very well be obtained from the woman's vagina after intercourse rather than through masturbation. But this would not make GIFT a more acceptable procedure. For the child would not be the fruit of the sexual act (through which the sperm was deposited in the vagina) but of the medical intervention of placing sperm and ova in one of the woman's fallopian tubes. In GIFT, how and when the sperm were obtained from the man makes no difference to the causal sequence leading to conception.

The situation is quite different in the case of the other procedure just described. Here the medical intervention does not involve the removal of the sperm from the woman's body (in order to reintroduce it on a later occasion). The medical intervention consists of using an instrument to help the sperm from the vagina through the cervix into the uterus, and to thus enable it to reach the site of fertilisation. The sexual act is an essential part of the sequence leading to conception. It, and not a medical intervention, initiates this sequence. This, then, is a procedure which married couples may justifiably be offered, since it is carried out in such a way that it does not bypass the normal conjugal act but merely helps the act to achieve the objective of fertilisation.

At present research is being undertaken in pursuit of a morally acceptable alternative to IVF and related procedures to overcome tubal blockage which cannot be surgically corrected. This alternative method is a way of overcoming tubal infertility without bypassing the sexual act. The technique involves transporting the ovum released during the *natural cycle* from the ovary to the uterus (or, possibly to the lower portion of the fallopian tube), there to be fertilised normally. Thus the ovum is collected, under ultrasound guidance, from the ovary by means of a fine tube passed through the vagina: as the tube is being withdrawn the ovum is deposited in the uterus. This technique respects the dignity of procreation by allowing the child to be begotten through sexual intercourse. It does not bypass the sexual act but makes it possible to achieve conception as a result of the sexual act. It also has the advantages that it does not require superovulation treatment and that it is a relatively simple procedure, requiring local anaesthesia only.

In short, not all forms of assisted reproduction are to be ruled out on the grounds that they fail to respect human dignity. There are modes of assisted reproduction which allow the child to be begotten in or through the conjugal sexual embrace, and so respect the personal integrity and the dignity of the couple and the child. Research aimed at perfecting such methods is to be welcomed, so that those couples who do not wish to resort to methods which are contrary to their human dignity may receive help to have the children they long for.

Glossary

Abortion: spontaneous or deliberately provoked loss of a fetus from the womb before it can survive independently.
Amniotic sac: membraneous sac of fluid surrounding the unborn child during pregnancy.
AID: artificial insemination by donor. *See* artificial insemination.
AIH: artificial insemination by husband. *See* artificial insemination.
Anaesthesia: procedure or medication that produces a loss of sensation.
Antibody: produced in the body to attack foreign substances such as bacteria or viruses; sometimes produced in either man or woman against sperm.
Artificial insemination: injection of semen into a woman's vagina or uterus.
Asthenospermia: loss or reduction of vitality of sperm in semen.
Azoospermia: failure to produce sperm.
Biopsy: surgical removal of cells or of a small piece of tissue for microscopic examination.
Capacitation: preparation of sperm enabling them to achieve fertilisation – a chemical process normally occurring as the sperm pass through the cervix and move on towards the site of fertilisation.

Caesarean section: surgical removal of the fetus from the womb via the abdominal wall.
Cervical mucus: mucus secreted by the cervix.
Cervix: neck of the uterus (womb).
Chromosome: chain-like microscopic bodies in the nucleus or centre of cells which contain the genes (the biological basis of heredity). The normal number of chromosomes in humans is 46.
Conception: the union of the ovum and the male sperm (also called fertilisation).
Conceptus: fertilised ovum.
Ectopic pregnancy: a dangerous condition in which the embryo starts growing outside the uterus, usually in the fallopian tube.
Embryo: conceptus from the time of fertilisation until some two months later, when it is sufficiently developed to be unmistakably human, that is, when the limbs and all the main organs are formed.
Embryo biopsy: removal of one or a few cells from the embryo for microscopic examination.
Embryogenesis: embryo development from the time of fertilisation until the end of the second month when the limbs and all the main organs are formed.
Endocrine glands: hormone-secreting glands.
Endometriosis: a condition involving misplaced endometrial tissue (lining of the womb) in the pelvic area. It may cause infertility.
Endometrium: lining of the uterus.
Extra-corporeal fertilisation: fertilisation outside the body.
Fallopian tube: tube connecting each ovary and the uterus.
Fetus: unborn child from the end of the second month until birth.
Fertilisation: the union of ovum and sperm (also called conception).

Fibroids: benign tumours of the uterus (womb), sometimes associated with infertility.
Gamete: germ cell, i.e. sperm or ovum.
Gene: the basic biological unit of heredity.
Genome: the total genetic content of an organism.
Gestation: the period of development of the unborn child in the womb from the time of fertilisation until birth.
GIFT: Gamete Intra-Fallopian Transfer, a procedure involving the transfer of ova and sperm to the fallopian tube where fertilisation may take place.
Gynaecology: the branch of medicine concerned with disorders of the female reproductive system.
Hormone: a chemical substance secreted into the blood by the endocrine glands in order to control bodily processes or stimulate other glands.
Identical twins: *See* monozygotic twins.
Immune system: the body's defence system against invading organisms such as bacteria and viruses.
Implantation: process whereby the embryo embeds itself in the lining of the uterus (womb).
Intra-uterine: within the uterus (womb).
In-vitro fertilisation (IVF): the technique of removing ova (or a single ovum) from a woman's body and fertilising them by mixing them with sperm in a glass dish with a view to transferring between one and three embryos to the uterus.
IVF: *See* In vitro fertilisation.
Laparoscope: the long narrow telescope which can be passed through the abdominal wall to inspect internal organs.
Laparoscopy: visualisation of internal organs by means of a laparoscope.
Menopause: the permanent cessation of menstrual periods.
Menstrual cycle: the regular monthly changes in the woman's body which control ovulation and menstruation.

Menstruation: the loss of blood from the vagina at the end of each menstrual cycle.

Monozygotic twins: twins originating from a single fertilised ovum.

Multiple pregnancy: a pregnancy with more than one child.

Non-therapeutic: non-healing.

Non-therapeutic research: research which is not aimed at benefiting the subject of the research but is undertaken for other purposes.

Obstetrics: the branch of medicine concerned with the pregnant woman and her unborn child until the time of birth and shortly after.

Oestrogen: the major female sex hormone.

Oligospermia: production of low numbers of sperm.

Ovarian follicle: a minute sac within the ovary containing the ovum, from which the ovum is released at ovulation.

Ovarian stimulation: hormone treatment with a view to inducing ovulation.

Ovary: female reproductive organ. There are two ovaries situated one on each side of the uterus.

Ovulation: the release of an ovum from an ovary.

Ovum, plural ova: female reproductive cell (egg).

Pelvic Inflammatory Disease: infection of the ovaries and fallopian tubes, which may cause infertility.

Pelvis: the bony basin containing the pelvic organs, e.g. the reproductive organs and the bladder.

Placenta: the spongy structure in the uterus (womb) through which the fetus gets its nourishment from the maternal blood via the umbilical cord.

Postcoital: after intercourse.

Premature birth: birth before the 37th week of pregnancy.

Prenatal diagnosis: diagnosis of fetal abnormality or illness.

Pre-implantation diagnosis: diagnosis of abnormality in the embryo in connection with artificial methods of conception and before implantation in the womb. *See* embryo biopsy.

Primary infertility: infertility in a couple – or a woman – with no previous child.

Primitive streak: longitudal axis in the developing embryo, which appears around the 14th day after fertilisation.

Procured abortion: abortion caused by drugs or surgical procedures.

Progesterone: one of the major female sex hormones.

PROST: Pronuclear Tubal Transfer; a procedure involving transfer of embryo(s) to the fallopian tubes.

Secondary infertility: infertility in a couple – or a woman – with a previous child.

Semen: fluid emitted from a man's penis at orgasm.

Seminal fluid: *See* semen.

Sex chromosome: an X or Y chromosome. Women have two X chromosomes and men have one X and one Y chromosome.

Subfertility: impaired fertility.

TEST: Tubal Embryo Transfer; a procedure involving the transfer of embryo(s) to the fallopian tubes.

Spina bifida: Congenital failure of the vertebrae or back bones to close, often resulting in hernial protrusion of the membranes of the spinal cord (open spina bifida), involving paralysis of the lower part of the body.

Super ovulation: hormone stimulation to induce the production of several ova in the same menstrual cycle.

Testis, plural *testes*: male reproductive organ which produces sperm.

Testosterone: the main male sex hormone.

Therapeutic: healing.

Therapeutic research: research aimed at benefiting the research subject.

Trimester: period of about three months. Pregnancy is divided into three trimesters.

Ultrasound scan: a technique for visualising internal organs by means of high-frequency (inaudible) sound waves.

Notes

1 *Donum Vitae* or *Instruction on Respect for Human Life in Its Origin and on the Dignity of Procreation*, English translation, Catholic Truth Society, London 1987, p. 36.
2 N Pfeffer and A Quick, *Infertility Services: A Desperate Case* (The Greater London Community Health Councils), London 1988, p. 15; J Yovich and G Grudzinskas, *The Management of Infertility: A Manual of Gamete Handling Procedures*, Oxford 1990, pp. 1–2.
3 J Yovich and G Grudzinskas, *op. cit.* p. 2.
4 N Pfeffer and A Quick, *op. cit.* p. 35; J Yovich and G Grudzinskas, *op. cit.* p. 16.
5 J Yovich and G Grudzinskas, *op. cit.* pp. 22–26; N Pfeffer and A Quick, *op. cit.* pp. 31, 37–38; G H Barker, *The New Fertility; A Guide to Modern Medical Treatment for Childless Couples*, London 1986, pp. 68–69, 72–74.
6 J Yovich and G Grudzinskas, *op. cit.* pp. 18–19.
7 G H Barker, *op. cit.* pp. 74–75, 112–114.
8 M C Wagner and P A Clair, 'Are *in vitro* fertilisation and embryo transfer of benefit to all?', *The Lancet*, 1989, vol. 2, pp. 1027–1029; *The Sixth Report of the Interim Licencing Authority (ILA) for Human in vitro Fertilisation and Embryology*, 1991, pp. 18–19, 23–25.
9 *Ibid.*

10 *Ibid.*
11 G H Barker, *op. cit.* p. 145; J Yovich and G Grudzinskas, *op. cit.* pp. 81–83.
12 G H Barker, *op. cit.*, p. 148.
13 J Yovich and G Grudzinskas, *op. cit.* pp. 70–75.
14 *Ibid.*
15 G H Barker, *op. cit.* p. 148.
16 G H Barker, *op. cit.* pp. 135–136; J Yovich and G Grudzinskas, *op. cit.* pp. 121–122.
17 G H Barker, *op. cit.* pp. 137–141; J Yovich and G Grudzinskas, *op. cit.* pp. 123–137.
18 It is not allowed to transfer more than three embryos to a woman in either IVF or GIFT. See *The Human Fertilisation and Embryology Act 1990*, Appendix 4, referring to The ILA (Interim Licencing Authority) Guidelines, para. 12. See also *Human Fertilisation & Embryology Authority: Code of Practice*, Part 7.6.
19 M C Wagner and P A Clair, *op. cit.*
20 Equally successful results (i.e. pregnancies) have been obtained without superovulation and by transferring one embryo only to the uterus. See H Foulot *et al.*, In vitro fertilisation without ovarian stimulation: a simplified protocol applied in 80 cycles', *Fertility and Sterility*, 1989, vol. 52, pp. 617–621.
21 *The Sixth Report of the Interim Licencing Authority*, 1991, p. 21.
22 Editorial, 'Preimplantation genetic diagnosis', *British Medical Journal*, 1990, vol. 301, pp. 894–895.
23 M C Wagner and P A Clair, *op. cit.*
24 *Ibid.*
25 *Ibid.*
26 A Fisher, *IVF: The Critical Issues*, Melbourne 1989, p. 71.
27 A success rate of 5.2–11.6 per cent live births per treatment cycle (depending on the size of the centre) is quoted in *The Sixth Report of The Interim Licensing Authority*, 1991, p. 21.

28 *The Human Fertilisation and Embryology Act 1990*, section 13 (5), states:
"A woman shall not be provided with treatment services unless account has been taken of the welfare of any child who may be born as a result of the treatment (including the need of that child for a father), and of any other child who may be affected by the birth."
Although the clause refers to the child's need of a father, it does not actually exclude single or lesbian women from treatment services.
29 J Yovich and G Grudzinskas, *op. cit.*, pp. 145–161.
30 *The Sixth Report of the Interim Licensing Authority*, 1991, p. 21.
31 J Yovich and G Grudzinskas, *op. cit.*, pp. 165–183.
32 J Yovich and G Grudzinskas, *op. cit.*, pp. 140, 161, 182, 197.
33 G Allen and Z Hrubec, 'The monozygotic twinning rate: is it really constant?', *Acta Geneticae Medicae et Gemellologicae Roma*, 1987, vol. 36, pp. 389–396.
34 J Yovich and G Grudzinskas, *op. cit.*, pp. 1–2.
35 F T Sai and K Newman, 'Ethics and Human Values in Family Planning: Africa Regional Perspective', *Ethics and Human Values in Family Planning: Conference Highlights, Papers and Discussion*, Proceedings of the 22nd CIOMS Conference, Bangkok, 19–24 June 1988, ed. Z Bankowski, J Barzelatto and A M Capron, p. 152.
36 J Yovich and G Grudzinskas, *op. cit.*, pp. 1–2.
37 *Ibid.*
38 *Ibid.*